DASH DIET
RECIPES

*Improving Health by Prevention with
Proper Nutrition*

SALLY MOORE

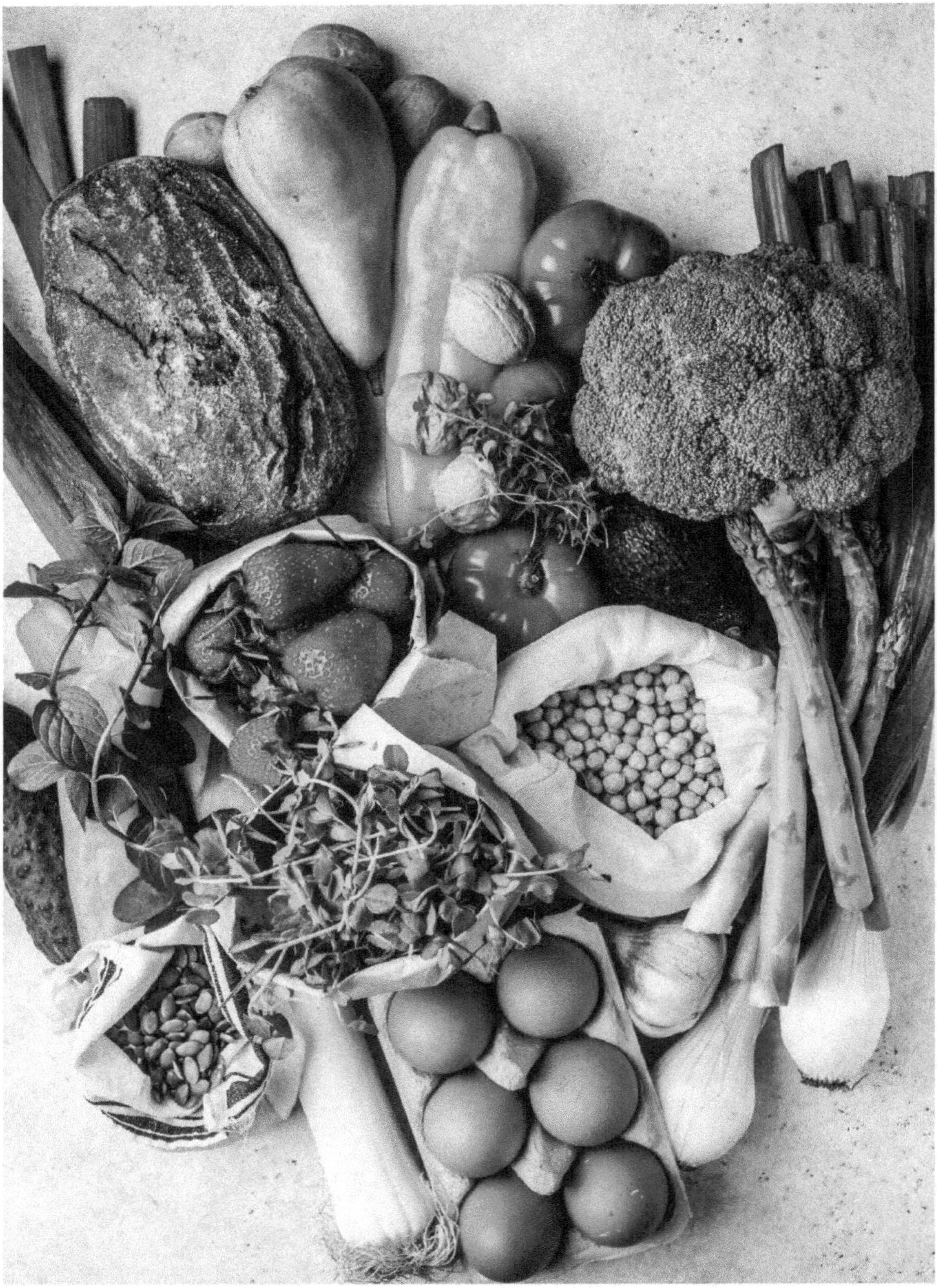

Table of Contents

Sommario

Introduction

What is the DASH diet?

The DASH diet, which is a dietary approach to stop hypertension, is promoted by the National Heart, Lung, and Blood Institute to achieve exactly that: stop or prevent hypertension, or high blood pressure.
It emphasizes the foods you've always eaten (fruits, vegetables, whole grains, lean proteins, and low-fat dairy products), which are rich in blood pressure-reducing nutrients like potassium, calcium, protein, and fiber.
DASH also avoids foods high in saturated fat, such as fatty meats, fatty dairy products, and tropical oils, as well as sugary drinks and sweets.
Following the DASH also involves limiting sodium to 2,300 milligrams per day, and those who follow it will eventually reduce sodium to about 1,500 milligrams.
The DASH diet is balanced and can be practiced long-term, which is the main reason why nutrition experts consider it the best diet ever along with the Mediterranean diet.

How does the DASH diet work?

Undertaking the DASH diet means not making drastic changes overnight.
Instead, start making small changes such as those you feel are more manageable.

The DASH diet involves a set number of daily servings of different food groups.

The number of servings you need may depend on the number of daily calories you need to consume.

Dash Diet Tips

Add a serving of vegetables at lunch and dinner.

Add a serving of fruit to your meals or as a snack.

Reduce your meat intake by eliminating it for at least 2 days a week.

Canned nuts are easy to use, but check to make sure they have no added sugars.

Use only half of your typical serving of butter, margarine, or salad dressings, and use low-fat or fat-free dressings.

Eat low-fat or skim dairy whenever you would normally use whole milk or cream.

Use herbs and spices that make food more flavorful without salt.

Snack on almonds or pecans instead of a bag of chips.

Substitute white flour for whole wheat whenever possible.

Read food labels so you can select low-sodium products.

Take a 15-minute walk after lunch or dinner (or both).

Enclosed in this book are several recipes selected to follow a diet with the Dash Diet criteria. Enjoy!

Breakfast

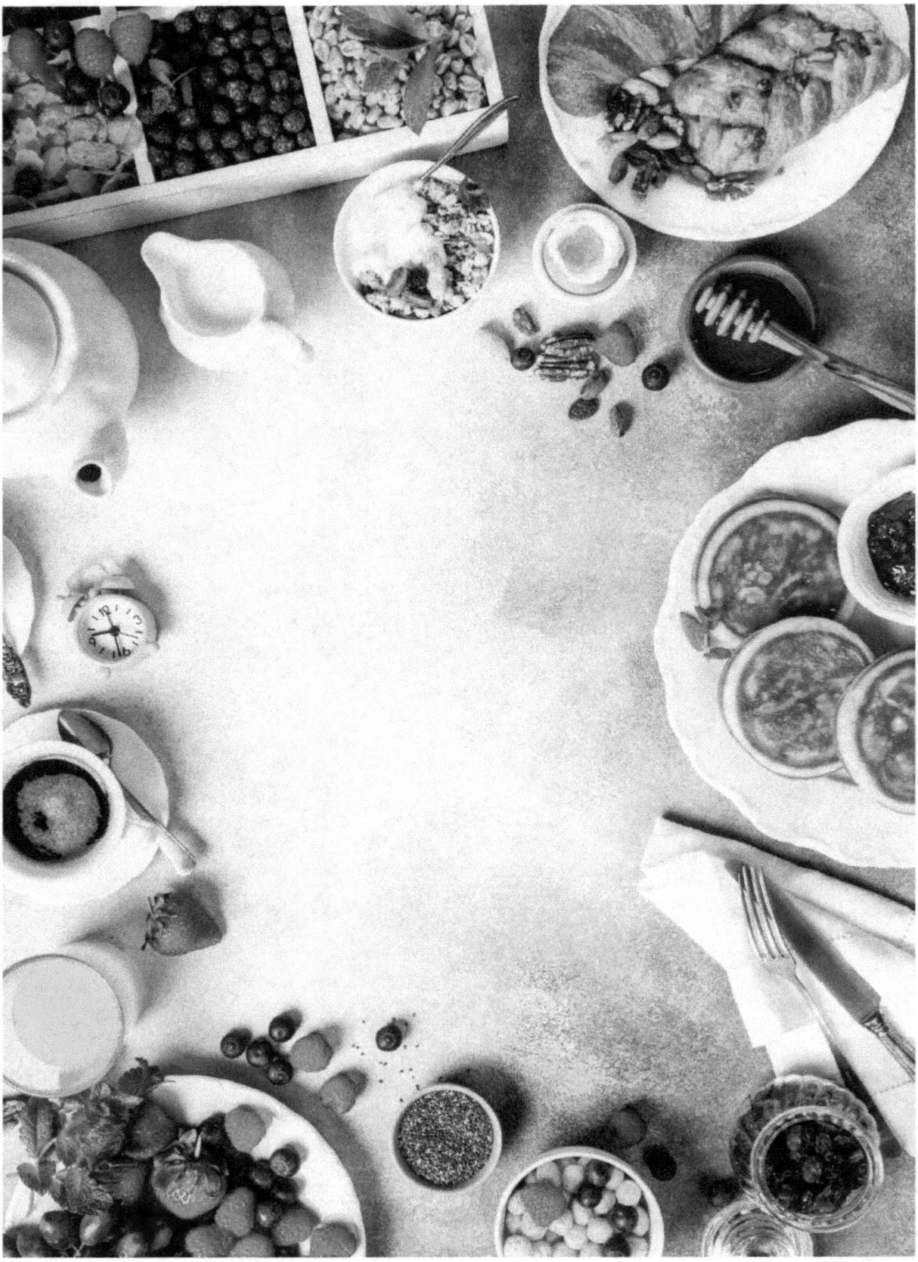

Banana And Walnuts Bowls

Preparation time: 10 minutes
Cooking time: 15 minutes
Servings: 4

Ingredients:
2 cups water
1 cup steel cut oats
1 cup almond milk
¼ cup walnuts, chopped
2 tablespoons chia seeds
2 bananas, peeled and mashed
1 teaspoon vanilla extract

Directions:
In a small pot, combine the water with the oats, milk, walnuts, chia seeds, bananas and vanilla, toss, bring to a simmer over medium heat, cook for 15 minutes, divide into bowls and serve for breakfast. Enjoy!

Nutrition: calories 162, fat 4, fiber 6, carbs 11, protein 4

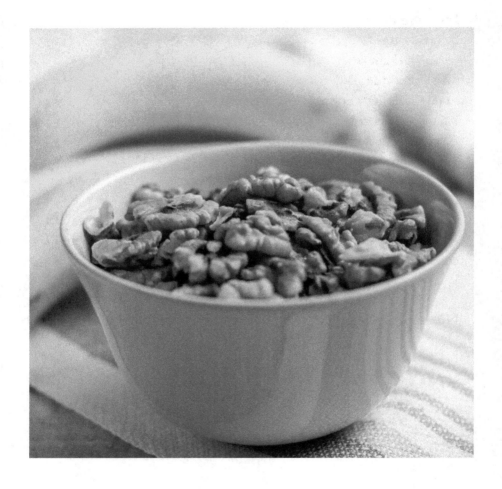

Parsley Omelet

Preparation time: 10 minutes
Cooking time: 6 minutes
Servings: 6

Ingredients:
2 tablespoons almond milk
A pinch of black pepper
6 eggs, whisked
2 tablespoons parsley, chopped
1 tablespoon low-fat cheddar cheese, shredded
2 teaspoons olive oil

Directions:
In a bowl, mix the eggs with the milk, black pepper, parsley and cheese and whisk well.
Add the eggs mix, spread into the pan, cook for 3 minutes, flip, cook for 3 minutes more on a heated pan with the oil over medium-high heat, divide between plates and serve for breakfast.
Enjoy!

Nutrition: calories 200, fat 4, fiber 6, carb 13, protein 9

Sweet Chia Bowls

Preparation time: 10 minutes
Cooking time: 2 hours
Servings: 4

Ingredients:
2 cups non-fat milk
1 cup brown rice
2 bananas, peeled and sliced
1 tablespoon maple syrup
2 tablespoons chia seeds
1 teaspoon sugar
1 teaspoon vanilla extract
1 teaspoon cinnamon powder

Directions:
1. In your slow cooker, combine the milk with the bananas, maple syrup and the other ingredients, put the lid on and cook on High for 2 hours.
2. Divide the mix into bowls and serve for breakfast.

Nutrition: Calories 321, Fat .3.5g, Cholesterol 3mg, Sodium 69mg, Carbohydrate 63.4g, Fiber 5.4g, Sugars 17.3g, Protein 9.3g, Potassium 577mg

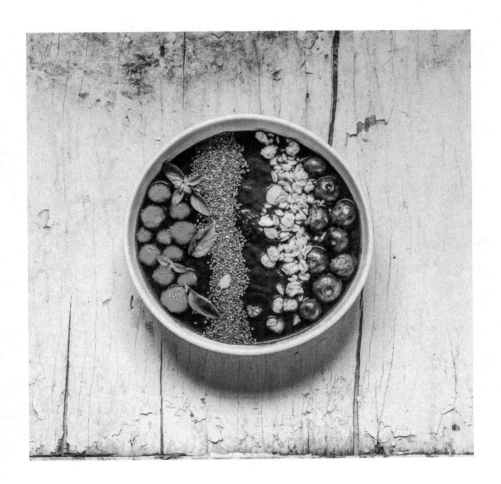

Spiced Oatmeal

Preparation time: 10 minutes
Cooking time: 9 hours
Servings: 4

Ingredients:
1 cup steel cut oats
2 tablespoons stevia
½ teaspoon cinnamon powder A pinch of cloves, ground
½ cup pumpkin puree
4 cups water
Olive oil cooking spray
½ cup fat-free milk
A pinch of nutmeg, ground
A pinch of allspice, ground
A pinch of ginger, ground

Directions:
Grease your slow cooker with the cooking spray, add the oats, the
pumpkin puree, water, milk, stevia, cinnamon, cloves, allspice, ginger
and nutmeg, cover and cook on Low for 9 hours.
Stir the oatmeal, divide it into bowls and serve.

Nutrition: Calories 100, Fat 1.5g, Cholesterol 1mg, Sodium 26mg,
Carbohydrate 25.5g, Fiber 3g, Sugars 2.7g, Protein 4g, Potassium
189mg

Creamy Oats, Greens & Blueberry Smoothie

Preparation time: 4 minutes
Cooking time: 0 minutes
Servings: 1

Ingredients:
1 c. cold
Fat-free milk
1 c. salad greens
1/2 c. fresh frozen blueberries
1/2 c. frozen cooked oatmeal
1 tbsp. sunflower seeds

Directions:
In a powerful blender, blend all ingredients until smooth and creamy.
Serve and enjoy.

Nutrition: Calories: 280, Fat: 6.8 g, Carbs: 44.0, g Protein: 14.0 g,
Sugars: 32 g, Sodium: 141%

Banana & Cinnamon Oatmeal

Preparation time: 5 minutes
Cooking time: 0 minutes
Servings: 6

Ingredients:
2 c. quick-cooking oats
4 c. Fat-free milk
1 tsp. ground cinnamon
2 chopped large ripe banana
4 tsps. Brown sugar
Extra ground cinnamon

Directions:
Place milk in a skillet and bring to boil. Add oats and cook over medium heat until thickened, for two to four minutes. Stir intermittently.
Add cinnamon, brown sugar and banana and stir to combine.
If you want, serve with the extra cinnamon and milk. Enjoy!

Nutrition: Calories: 215, Fat: 2 g, Carbs: 42 g, Protein: 10 g, Sugars: 1 g, Sodium: 40%

Basil and Tomato Baked Eggs

Preparation time: 10 minutes
Cooking Time: 15 minutes
Serving: 2

Ingredients:
1/2 garlic clove, minced
1/2 cup canned tomatoes
¼ cup fresh basil leaves, roughly chopped
1/4 teaspoon chili powder
1/2 tablespoon olive
oil 2 whole eggs
Pepper to taste

Directions:
Preheat your oven to 375 degrees F.
Take a small baking dish and grease with olive oil.
Add garlic, basil, tomatoes chili, olive oil into a dish and stir. Crack eggs into a dish, keeping space between the two. Sprinkle the whole dish with sunflower seeds and pepper.
Place in oven and cook for 12 minutes until eggs are set and tomatoes are bubbling.
Serve with basil on top. Enjoy!

Nutrition: Calories: 235, Fat: 16g, Carbohydrates: 7g, Protein: 14g

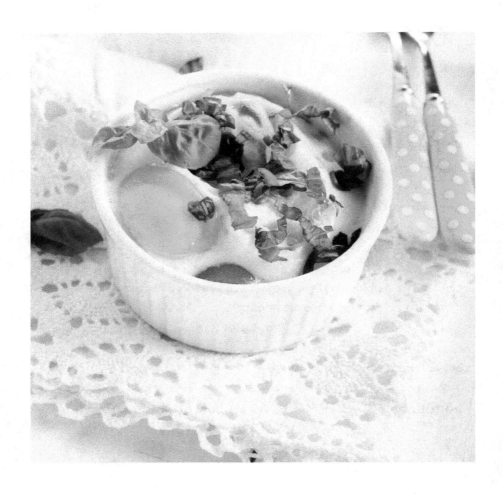

Cool Mushroom Munchies

Preparation time: 5 minutes
Cooking Time: 10 minutes
Serving: 2

Ingredients:
4 Portobello mushroom caps
3 tablespoons coconut aminos
2 tablespoons sesame oil
1 tablespoon fresh ginger, minced
1 small garlic clove, minced

Directions:
Set your broiler to low, keeping the rack 6 inches from the heating source.
Wash mushrooms under cold water and transfer them to a baking sheet (top side down).
Take a bowl and mix in sesame oil, garlic, coconut aminos, ginger and pour the mixture over the mushrooms tops .
Cook for 10 minutes. Serve and enjoy!

Nutrition: Calories: 196, Fat: 14g, Carbohydrates: 14g, Protein: 7g

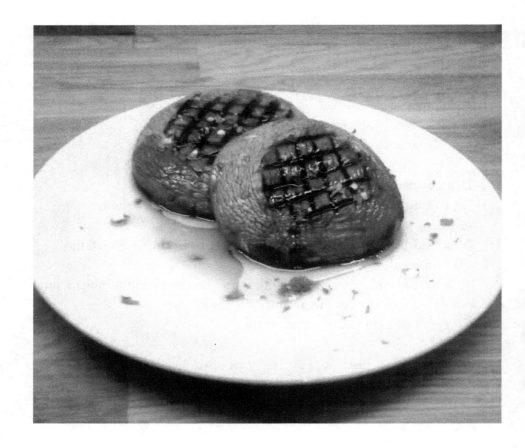

Soups

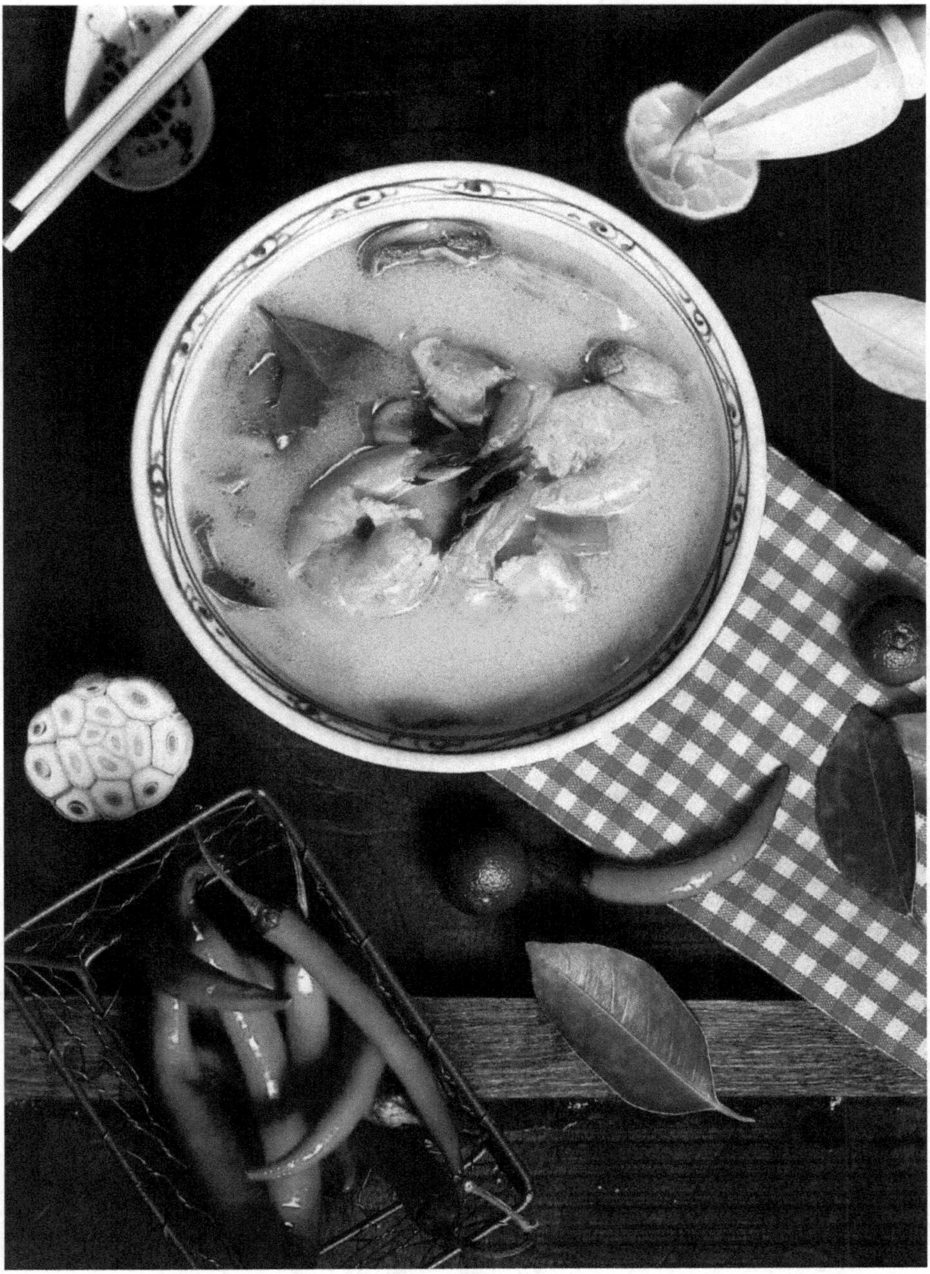

Taco Soup

Preparation time: 15 minutes
Cooking time: 8 hours
Servings: 6

Ingredients:
1-pound ground turkey breast
1 onion, chopped
1 can tomatoes and green chilis, with their juice
6 cups Poultry Broth or store-bought
1 teaspoon chili powder
1 teaspoon ground cumin
½ teaspoon of sea salt
¼ cup chopped fresh cilantro Juice of 1 lime
½ cup grated low-fat Cheddar cheese

Directions:
Crumble the turkey into the slow cooker. Add the onion, tomatoes, green chilis (with their juice), broth, chili powder, cumin, and salt. Cover and cook on low within 8 hours. Stir in the cilantro and lime juice. Serve garnished with the cheese.

Nutrition: Calories: 281, Fat: 10g, Carbohydrates: 20g, Fiber: 5g, Protein: 30g, Sodium: 470 mg

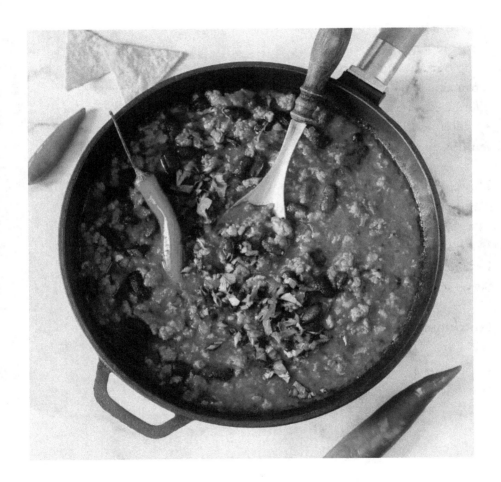

Minty Avocado Soup

Preparation time: 10 minutes+ Chill time
Cooking Time: Nil
Serving: 4

Ingredients:
1 avocado, ripe
1 cup coconut almond milk, chilled
2 romaine lettuce leaves
20 mint leaves, fresh
1 tablespoon lime juice
Sunflower seeds, to taste

Directions:
Turn on your slow cooker and add all the ingredients into it.
Mix them in a food processor.
Make a smooth mixture.
Let it chill for 10 minutes.
Serve and enjoy!

Nutrition: Calories: 280, Fat: 26g, Carbohydrates: 12g, Protein: 4g

Celery Cream Soup

Preparation time: 10 minutes
Cooking Time: 25 minutes
Servings: 1

Ingredients:
2 cups celery stalk, chopped
1 shallot, chopped
1 potato, chopped
4 cups low-sodium vegetable stock
1 tablespoon margarine
1 teaspoon white pepper

Directions:
Melt the margarine in the saucepan, add shallot, and celery stalk. Cook the vegetables for 5 minutes. Stir them occasionally.
After this, add vegetable stock and potato.
Simmer the soup for 15 minutes.
Blend the soup tilly you get the creamy texture and sprinkle with white pepper.
Simmer it for 5 minutes more.

Nutrition: 88 calories, 2.3g protein, 13.3g carbohydrates, 3g fat, 2.9g fiber, 0mg cholesterol, 217mg sodium, 449mg potassium.

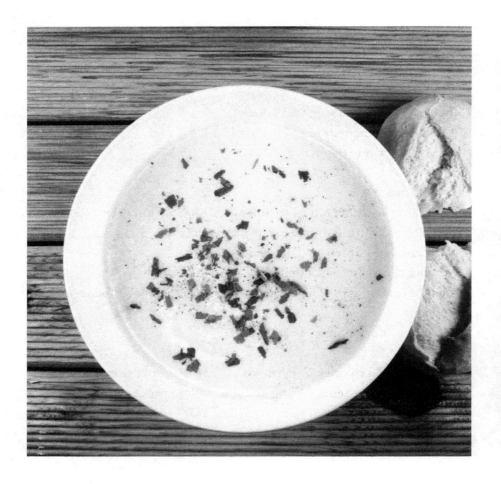

Cauliflower Soup

Preparation time: 10 minutes
Cooking Time: 20 minutes
Servings: 2

Ingredients:
1 cup cauliflower, chopped
¼ cup potato, chopped
1 cup skim milk
1 cup of water
1 teaspoon ground coriander
1 teaspoon margarine

Directions:
Put cauliflower and potato in the saucepan.
Add water and boil the ingredients for 15 minutes.
Then add ground coriander and margarine.
With the help of the immersion blender, blend the soup until smooth.
Add skim milk and stir well.

Nutrition: 82 calories, 5.2g protein,10.3g carbohydrates, 2g fat, 1.5g fiber, 2mg cholesterol, 106mg sodium, 384mg potassium.

Cauliflower Butternut Soup

Preparation time: 5 minutes
Cooking Time: 25 minutes
Servings: 6

Ingredients:
1 diced onion
2-3 cloves minced garlic
1-pound frozen butternut squash
1 teaspoon paprika
½ teaspoon red pepper flakes
½ cup cream
1-pound frozen cauliflower
2 cups vegetable broth
1 teaspoon diced thyme
¼ teaspoon sea salt
2 teaspoons oil for sautéing
topping such as cheddar cheese, crumbled bacon, sour cream, chives, cheddar, and crumbled bacon

Directions:
Heat oil up in pressure cooker, and sauté onion, adding garlic to mixture. Add the cauliflower, broth, spices, and butternut, and from there, mix it together.
Cook on manual high for 5 minutes, and natural pressure release, and from there, blend it through an immersion blender, and then serve!

Nutrition: Calories: 100, Fat: 3g, Carbs: 16g, Net Carbs: 13g, Protein: 5g, Fiber: 3g

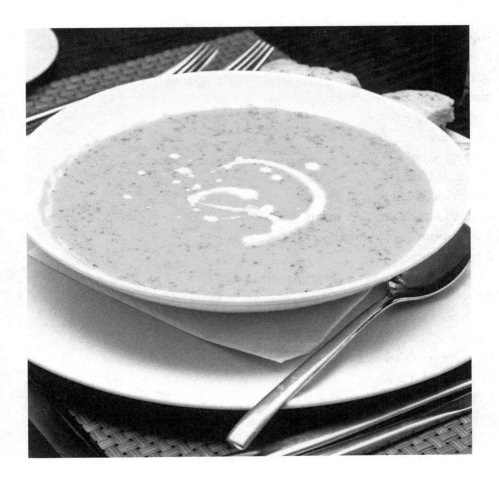

Vegetable Beef Stew

Preparation time: 20 minutes
Cooking Time: 60 minutes
Servings: 6

Ingredients:
2 pounds cubed beef chuck and 1 tablespoon olive oil
½ cup peeled turnip,
diced ¼ cup rolled carrots
¼ cup sliced celery
¼ cup cut string beans
2 cloves sliced garlic
½ cup red wine
¾ cup diced red onions
4 cups low-sodium beef broth
2 tablespoons red tomato paste
2 tablespoons beef base
1 tablespoon porcini mushroom powder
2 cloves
2 teaspoons gelatin powder
2 bay leaves
½ teaspoon dried marjoram
Salt and pepper for taste
1 teaspoon rubbed thyme
4 tablespoons cooking butter

Directions:

Trim beef chuck of silver skin and fat and cube it, prepare veggies as well. Turn on sauté mode and brown beef in batches, and from there, you add the rest of the ingredients and then stir together. Press soup button, and let it natural pressure release, when finished, you can adjust with seasonings.

Nutrition: Calories: 321, Fat: 15g, Carbs: 10g, Net Carbs: 7g, Protein: 33g, Fiber: 3g

Cauliflower Butternut Soup

Preparation time: 5 minutes
Cooking Time: 25 minutes
Servings: 6

Ingredients:
1 diced onion
2-3 cloves minced garlic
1-pound frozen butternut squash
1 teaspoon paprika
½ teaspoon red pepper flakes
½ cup cream
1-pound frozen cauliflower
2 cups vegetable broth
1 teaspoon diced thyme
¼ teaspoon sea salt
2 teaspoons oil for sautéing
topping such as cheddar cheese, crumbled bacon, sour cream, chives, cheddar, and crumbled bacon

Directions:
Heat oil up in pressure cooker, and sauté onion, adding garlic to mixture. Add the cauliflower, broth, spices, and butternut, and from there, mix it together.
Cook on manual high for 5 minutes, and natural pressure release, and from there, blend it through an immersion blender, and then serve!

Nutrition: Calories: 100, Fat: 3g, Carbs: 16g, Net Carbs: 13g, Protein: 5g, Fiber: 3g

Vegetable Beef Stew

Preparation time: 20 minutes
Cooking Time: 60 minutes
Servings: 6

Ingredients:

2 pounds cubed beef chuck and 1 tablespoon olive oil
½ cup peeled turnip, diced ¼ cup rolled carrots
¼ cup sliced celery ¼ cup cut string beans 2 cloves sliced garlic
½ cup red wine
¾ cup diced red onions
4 cups low-sodium beef broth
2 tablespoons red tomato paste
2 tablespoons beef base
1 tablespoon porcini mushroom powder
2 cloves
2 teaspoons gelatin powder
2 bay leaves
½ teaspoon dried marjoram Salt and pepper for taste
1 teaspoon rubbed thyme
4 tablespoons cooking butter

Directions:

Trim beef chuck of silver skin and fat and cube it, prepare veggies as well. Turn on sauté mode and brown beef in batches, and from there, you add the rest of the ingredients and then stir together. Press soup button, and let it natural pressure release, when finished, you can adjust with seasonings.

Nutrition: Calories: 321, Fat: 15g, Carbs: 10g, Net Carbs: 7g, Protein: 33g, Fiber: 3g

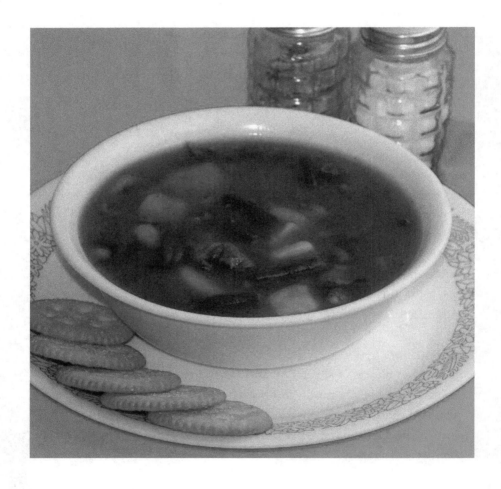

Poultry

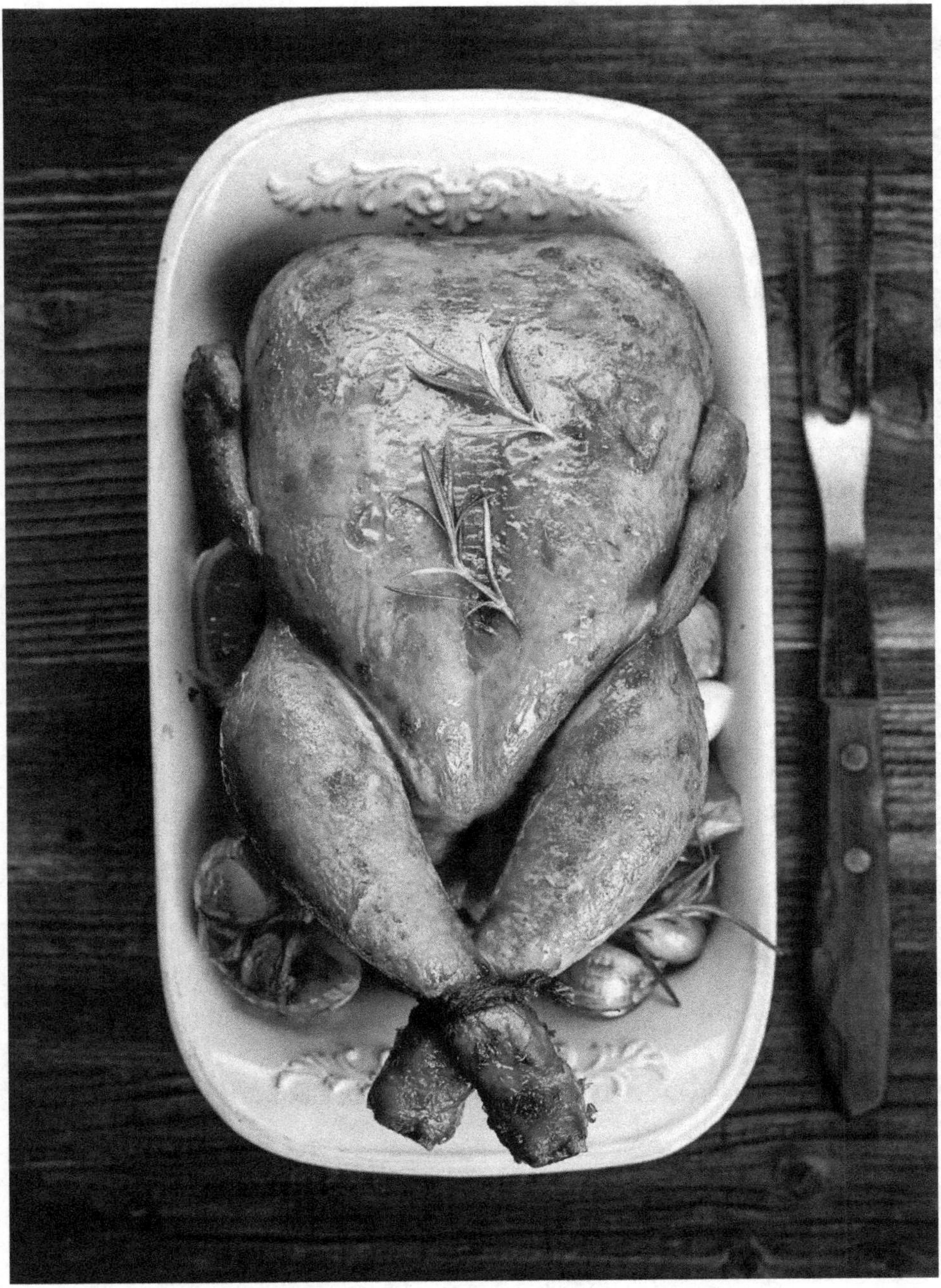

Chicken with Potatoes Olives & Sprouts

Preparation time: 15 minutes
Cooking time: 35 minutes
Servings: 4

Ingredients:
1 lb. chicken breasts, skinless, boneless, and cut into pieces
¼ cup olives, quartered
1 tsp oregano
1 ½ tsp Dijon mustard
1 lemon juice
1/3 cup vinaigrette dressing
1 medium onion, diced
3 cups potatoes cut into pieces
4 cups Brussels sprouts, trimmed and quartered
¼ tsp pepper
¼ tsp salt

Directions:
1. Warm-up oven to 400 F. Place chicken in the center of the baking tray, then place potatoes, sprouts, and onions around the chicken.
2. In a small bowl, mix vinaigrette, oregano, mustard, lemon juice, and salt and pour over chicken and veggies. Sprinkle olives and season with pepper.
3. Bake in preheated oven for 20 minutes. Transfer chicken to a plate. Stir the vegetables and roast for 15 minutes more. Serve and enjoy.

Nutrition: Calories: 397, Fat: 13g, Protein: 38.3g, Carbs: 31.4g, Sodium 175 mg

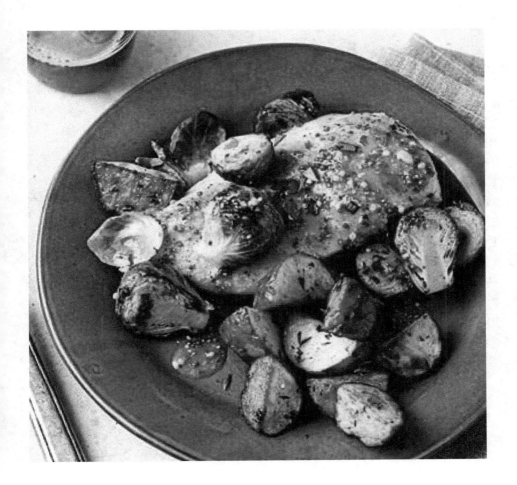

Pear Chicken Casserole

Preparation time: 10 minutes
Cooking time: 5 minutes
Servings: 8

Ingredients:
2 tablespoons olive oil
2 pounds chicken breasts, skinless and boneless
2 carrots, chopped
Black pepper to the taste
1 yellow onion, chopped
1 teaspoon Cajun seasoning
¼ cup flour
½ cup orange juice
1 can low sodium chicken stock
1 cup peas
½ cup parsley, chopped
2 tablespoons dill, chopped
½ cup fat free yogurt
2 and ½ cups cornflakes

Directions:

Put water in a pot, add chicken, bring to a boil over medium heat, simmer for 10 minutes, drain and leave aside for now. Heat up a pan with the oil over medium high heat, add onion, carrots and pepper, stir and cook for 10 minutes. Add Cajun seasoning and flour, stir and cook for 1 minute. Add stock and orange juice stirring all the time and bring to a boil. Add chicken, dill, peas and half of the parsley, stir and take off heat. Add yogurt, stir, transfer everything to a baking dish, introduce in the oven at 375 degrees F and bake for 15 minutes. Meanwhile, in a bowl, mix cornflakes with the rest of the parsley and stir. Take chicken out of the oven, sprinkle cornflakes all over, introduce in the oven again and bake for 6 more minutes. Take dish out of the oven, leave aside for 10 minutes, divide between plates and serve.

Nutrition: Calories 143, Protein 102g, Carbohydrates 66g, Fat 18g, Sodium 97mg

Chicken Divan

Preparation time: 15 minutes
Cooking time: 30 minutes
Servings: 4

Ingredients:
1/2-pound cooked chicken, boneless, skinless, diced in bite-size pieces
1 cup broccoli, cooked, diced into bite-size pieces 1 cup extra sharp cheddar cheese, grated 1 can mushroom soup
½ cup of water
1 cup croutons

Directions:
Warm oven to 350 F. In a large pot, heat the soup and water. Add the chicken, broccoli, and cheese. Combine thoroughly. Pour into a greased baking dish. Place the croutons over the mixture. Bake within 30 minutes or until the casserole is bubbling, and the croutons are golden brown.

Nutrition: Calories 380, Protein 25g, Carbohydrates 10g, Sugars 1g, Fat 22g, Sodium 397mg

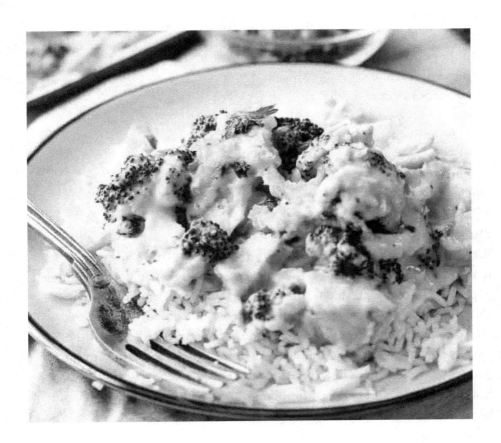

Honey Spiced Cajun Chicken

Preparation time: 15 minutes
Cooking time: 20 minutes
Servings: 4

Ingredients:
2 chicken breasts, skinless, boneless
1 Tablespoon butter or margarine
1 pound of linguini
3 large mushrooms, sliced
1 large tomato, diced
2 Tablespoons regular mustard
4 Tablespoons honey
3 ounces low-fat table cream
Parsley, roughly chopped

Directions:
Wash and dry the chicken breasts. Warm 1 tablespoon of butter or margarine in a large pan. Add the chicken breasts. Season with salt and pepper. Cook on each side 6 – 10 minutes, until cooked thoroughly. Pull the chicken breasts from the pan. Set aside. Cook the linguine as stated to instructions on the package in a large pot. Save 1 cup of the pasta water. Drain the linguine. Add the mushrooms, tomatoes to the pan from cooking the chicken. Heat until they are tender. Add the honey, mustard, and cream. Combine thoroughly. Add the chicken and linguine to the pan. Stir until coated. Garnish with parsley. Serve immediately.

Nutrition: Calories 112, Protein 12g, Carbohydrates 56g, Fat 20g, Sodium 158mg

Turkey Breast with Tomato-Olive Salsa

Preparation Time: 20 minutes
Cooking Time: 10 minutes
Servings: 4

Ingredients:
For turkey:
 4 boneless turkey. Skinned.
3 tablespoons olive oil
Salt
Pepper
 For salsa:
 6 chopped tomatoes
1/2 diced onions
5 ounces of pitted and chopped olives
2 crushed garlic cloves
2 tablespoons of chopped basil
1 large diced jalapeno
Pepper
Salt

Directions:
In a bowl, put salt, pepper, and three spoons of oil, mix and coat the turkey with this mixture. Place it on a preheated grill and grill for ten minutes. In another bowl, mix garlic, olives, tomatoes, pepper, and drop the rest of the oil. Sprinkle salt and toss. Serve this salsa with turkey is warm.

Nutrition: Calories: 387, Fat: 12.5g, Fiber: 8.4g, Carbohydrates:3.1g, Protein: 18.6g

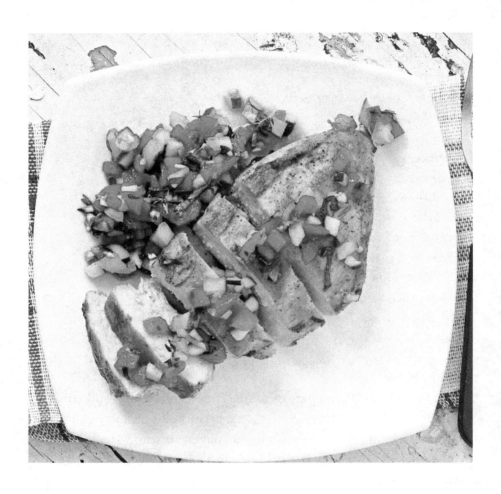

Tuscan Chicken

Preparation Time: 15 minutes
Cooking Time: 15 minutes
Servings: 6

Ingredients:
11/2 pounds chicken breasts, pasteurized, skinless, thinly sliced
1/2 cup sun-dried tomatoes
1 cup spinach, chopped
1 teaspoon garlic powder
teaspoon Italian seasoning
tablespoons avocado oil
1/2 cup grated parmesan cheese
1 cup heavy cream,
full-fat 1/2 cup chicken broth, pasteurized

Directions:
Take a large skillet pan, place it over medium-high heat, add oil, and when hot, add chicken and then cook for 3–5 minutes per side until golden brown. Add garlic powder, Italian seasoning, and cheese into the pan, pour in the broth and cream, and then whisk until combined. Switch heat to medium-high, cook the sauce for 2 minutes until it begins to thicken, then add tomatoes and spinach and simmer until spinach leaves begin to wilt. Return chicken to the pan, toss until mixed, and cook for 2 minutes until hot. Serve chicken with cooked Keto pasta, such as zucchini noodles.

Nutrition: Calories: 390, Fat: 16.1g, Fiber: 12.8g, Carbohydrates: 3g, Protein: 19g

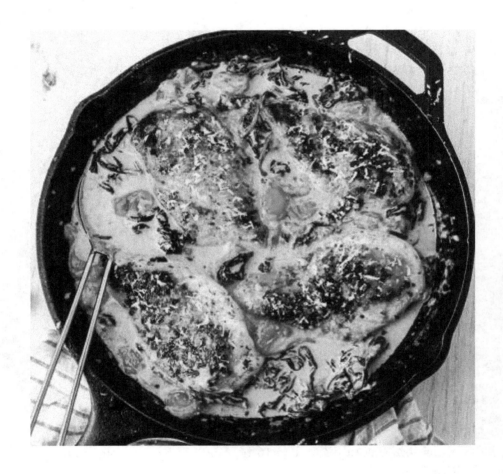

Cheesy Roasted Chicken

Preparation Time: 15 minutes
Cooking Time: 10 minutes
Servings: 6

Ingredients:
3 cups of chopped roasted chicken
2 cups of shredded cheddar cheese
cups white of shredded cheddar cheese
cups of shredded parmesan cheese

Directions:
Oven: 350F
Be sure to rub butter or to spray with non-stick cooking spray.
In a bowl, put in all the cheese and mix well.
Microwave the cheese till it melts
Put in the chicken and toss thoroughly.
Put two tablespoons of the cheese chicken combo in a pile on the baking sheet. Be sure to leave space between piles.
Bake for 4-6 minutes. The moment they turn golden brown at the edges, take them off.
Serve hot.

Nutrition: Calories: 387, Fat: 19.5g, Fiber: 4.1g, Carbohydrates:3.9g, Protein: 14.5g

Chicken Mélange

Preparation time: 15 minutes
Cooking time: 35 minutes
Servings: 3

Ingredients:
2 ounces (57 g) bacon, diced
¾ pound (340 g) whole chicken, boneless and chopped
½ medium-sized leek, chopped
1 teaspoon ginger garlic paste
1 teaspoon poultry seasoning mix
Sea salt, to taste
1 bay leaf
1 thyme sprig
1 rosemary sprig
cup chicken broth
½ cup cauliflower, chopped into small florets
vine-ripe tomatoes, puréed

Directions:
Heat a medium-sized pan over medium-high heat; once hot, fry the
bacon until it is crisp or about 3 minutes. Add in the chicken and cook
until it is no longer pink; reserve.
Then, sauté the leek until tender and fragrant. Stir in the ginger garlic
paste, poultry seasoning mix, salt, bay leaf, thyme, and rosemary.
Pour in the chicken broth and reduce the heat to medium; let it cook
for 15 minutes, stirring periodically.
Add in the cauliflower and tomatoes along with the reserved bacon and
chicken. Decrease the temperature to simmer and let it cook for a
further 15 minutes or until warmed through. Bon appétit!

Nutrition: calories: 353, fat: 14.4g, protein: 44.1g, carbs: 5.9g,
net carbs: 3.5g, fiber: 2.4g

Seafood

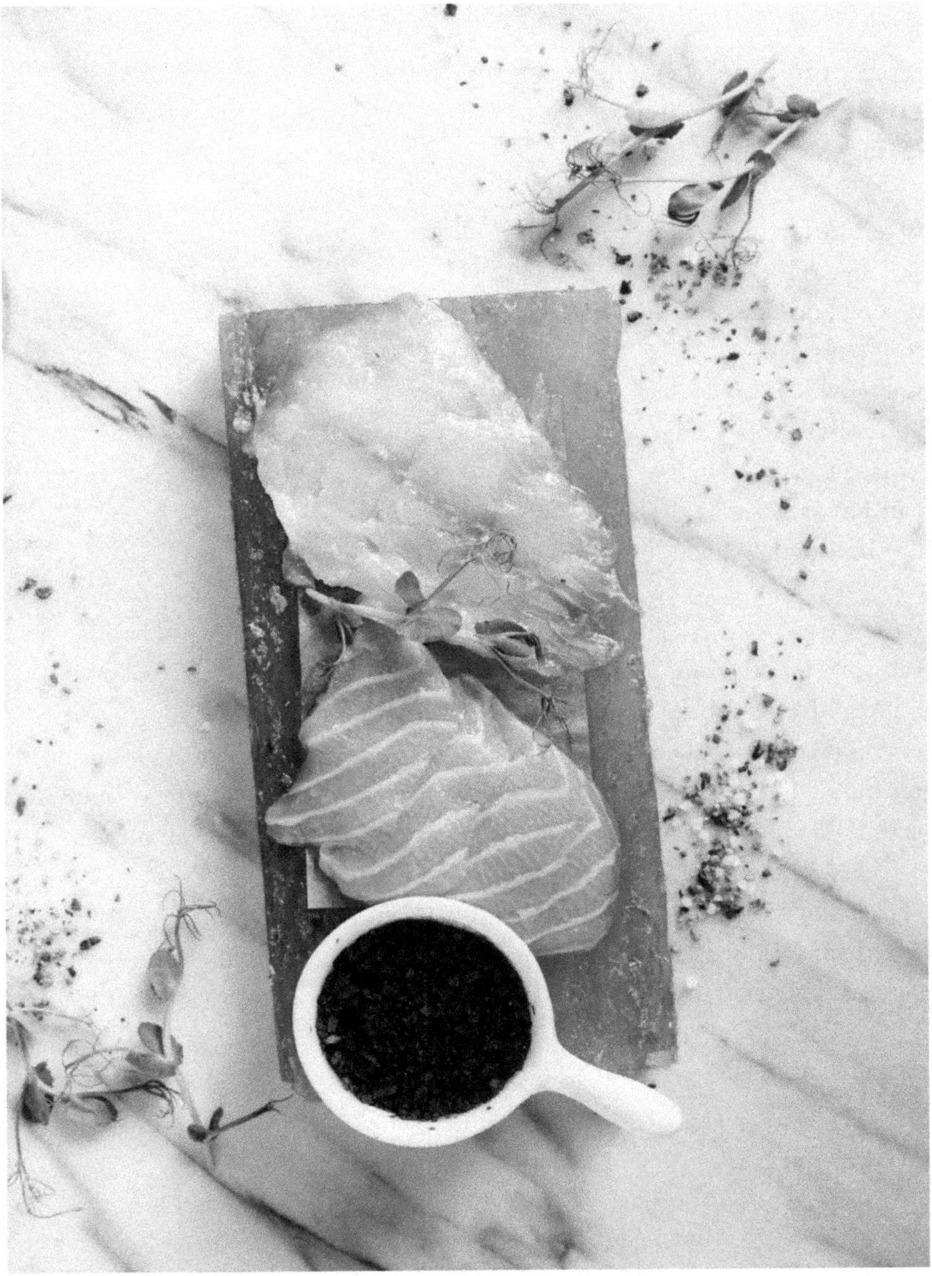

The OG Tuna Sandwich

Preparation time: 15 minutes
Cooking Time: 5 minutes
Servings: 2

Ingredients:
30 g olive oil
1 peeled and diced medium cucumber
2 ½ g pepper
4 whole wheat bread slices
85 g diced onion
2 ½ g salt
1 can flavored tuna
85 g shredded spinach

Directions:
Grab your blender and add the spinach, tuna, onion, oil, salt and pepper in, and pulse for about 10 to 20 seconds. In the meantime, toast your bread and add your diced cucumber to a bowl, which you can pour your tuna mixture in. Carefully mix and add the mixture to the bread once toasted. Slice in half and serve, while storing the remaining mixture in the fridge.

Nutrition: Calories: 302, Fat: 5.8 g, Carbs: 36.62 g, Protein: 28 g, Sugars: 3.22 g, Sodium: 445 mg

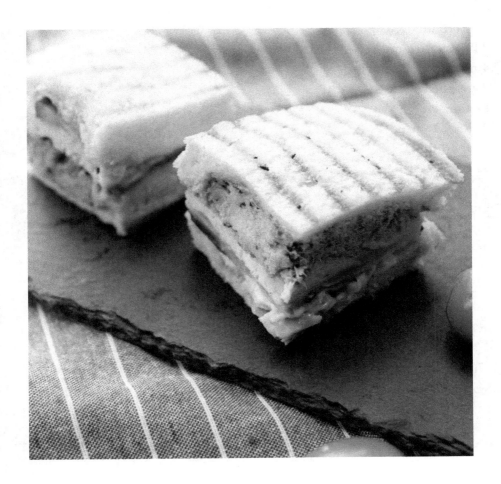

Easy to Understand Mussels

Preparation time: 10 minutes
Cooking Time: 10 minutes
Servings: 2

Ingredients:
2 lbs. cleaned mussels
4 minced garlic cloves
2 chopped shallots
Lemon and parsley
2 tbsps. Butter
½ c. broth
½ c. white wine

Directions:
Clean the mussels and remove the beard. Discard any mussels that do not close when tapped against a hard surface. Set your pot to Sauté mode and add chopped onion and butter. Stir and sauté onions. Add garlic and cook for 1 minute. Add broth and wine. Lock up the lid and cook for 5 minutes on HIGH pressure Release the pressure naturally over 10 minutes Serve with a sprinkle of parsley and enjoy!

Nutrition: Calories: 286, Fat: 14 g, Carbs: 12 g, Protein: 28 g, Sugars: 0 g. Sodium: 314 mg

Inspiring Cajun Snow Crab

Preparation time: 10 minutes
Cooking Time: 10 minutes
Serving: 2

Ingredients:
1 lemon, fresh and quartered
3 tablespoons Cajun seasoning
2 bay leaves
4 snow crab legs, precooked and defrosted
Golden ghee

Directions:
Take a large pot and fill it about halfway with sunflower seeds and water.
Bring the water to a boil.
Squeeze lemon juice into the pot and toss in remaining lemon quarters.
Add bay leaves and Cajun seasoning.
Season for 1 minute.
Add crab legs and boil for 8 minutes (make sure to keep them submerged the whole time).
Melt ghee in microwave and use as dipping sauce, enjoy!

Nutrition: Calories: 643, Fat: 51g, Carbohydrates: 3g, Protein: 41g

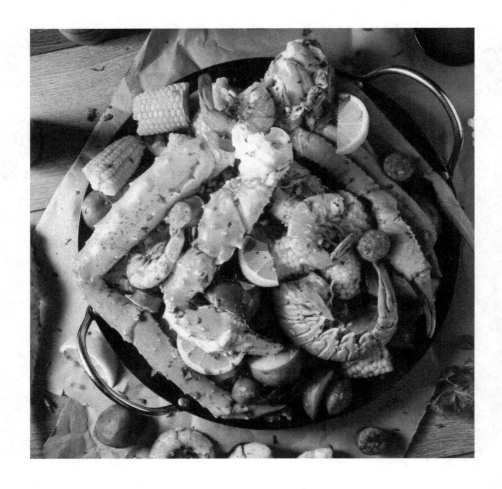

Grilled Lime Shrimp

Preparation time: 25 minutes
Cooking Time: 5 minutes
Serving: 8

Ingredients:
1 pound medium shrimp, peeled and deveined
1 lime, juiced
½ cup olive oil
3 tablespoons Cajun seasoning

Directions:
Take a re-sealable zip bag and add lime juice, Cajun seasoning, olive oil.
Add shrimp and shake it well, let it marinate for 20 minutes.
Preheat your outdoor grill to medium heat.
Lightly grease the grate.
Remove shrimp from marinade and cook for 2 minutes per side. Serve and enjoy!

Nutrition: Calories: 188, Fat: 3g, Net Carbohydrates: 1.2g, Protein: 13g

Salmon with Mushroom

Preparation time: 30 minutes
Cooking time: 10 minutes
Servings: 4

Ingredients:
8 ounces salmon fillets, boneless
2 tablespoons olive oil
Black pepper to the taste
2 ounces white mushrooms, sliced
½ shallot, chopped
2 tablespoons balsamic vinegar
2 teaspoons mustard
3 tablespoons parsley, chopped

Directions:
Brush salmon fillets with 1 tablespoon olive oil, season with black pepper, place on preheated grill over medium heat, cook for 4 minutes on each side and divide between plates.
Heat up a pan with the rest of the oil over medium-high heat, add mushrooms, shallot and some black pepper, stir and cook for 5 minutes.
Add the mustard, the vinegar and the parsley, stir, cook for 2-3 minutes more, add over the salmon and serve.
Enjoy!

Nutrition: calories 220, fat 4, fiber 8, carbs 6, protein 1

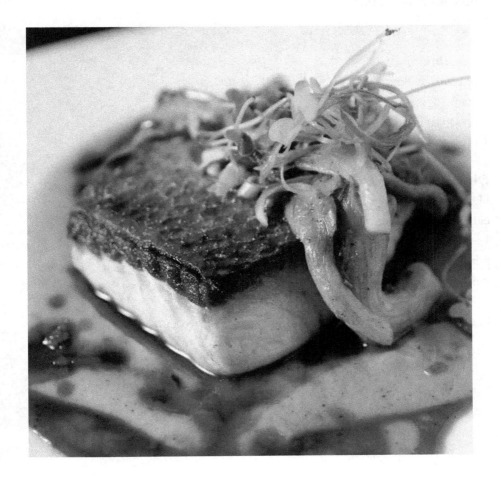

Scallops and Strawberry Mix

Preparation time: 10 minutes
Cooking time: 6 minutes
Servings: 2

Ingredients:
4 ounces scallops
½ cup Pico de gallo
½ cup strawberries, chopped
1 tablespoon lime juice Black pepper to the taste

Directions:
Heat up a pan over medium heat, add scallops, cook for 3 minutes on each side and take off heat,
In a bowl, mix strawberries with lime juice, Pico de gallo, scallops and pepper, toss and serve cold.
Enjoy!

Nutrition: calories 169, fat 2, fiber 2, carbs 8, protein 13

Simple Sautéed Garlic and Parsley Scallops

Preparation time: 5 minutes
Cooking Time: 25 minutes
Serving: 4

Ingredients:
8 tablespoons almond butter
2 garlic cloves, minced
16 large sea scallops
Sunflower seeds and pepper to taste
1 ½ tablespoons olive oil

Directions:
Seasons scallops with sunflower seeds and pepper.
Take a skillet, place it over medium heat, add oil and let it heat up.
Sauté scallops for 2 minutes per side, repeat until all scallops are cooked.
Add almond butter to the skillet and let it melt.
Stir in garlic and cook for 15 minutes.
Return scallops to skillet and stir to coat.
Serve and enjoy!

Nutrition: Calories: 417, Fat: 31g, Net Carbohydrates: 5g, Protein: 29g

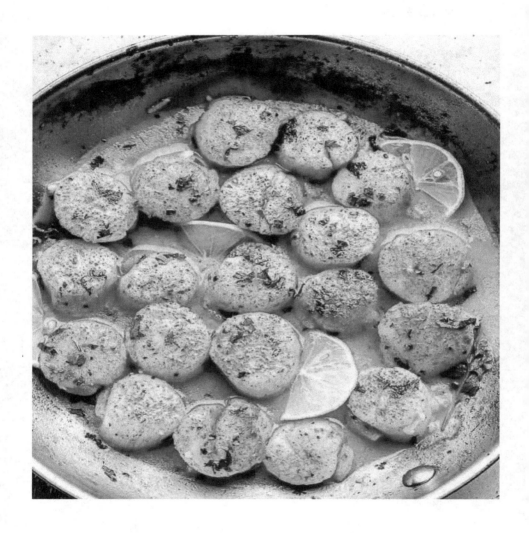

Salmon and Cucumber Platter

Preparation time: 10 minutes
Cooking Time: Nil
Serving: 4

Ingredients:
2 cucumbers, cubed
2 teaspoons fresh squeezed lemon juice
4 ounces non-fat yogurt
1 teaspoon lemon zest, grated
Pepper to taste
2 teaspoons dill, chopped
8 ounces smoked salmon, flaked

Directions:
Take a bowl and add cucumbers, lemon juice, lemon zest, pepper, dill, salmon, yogurt and toss well.
Serve cold.
Enjoy!

Nutrition: Calories: 242, Fat: 3g, Carbohydrates: 3g, Protein: 3g

Vegetarian and Vegan

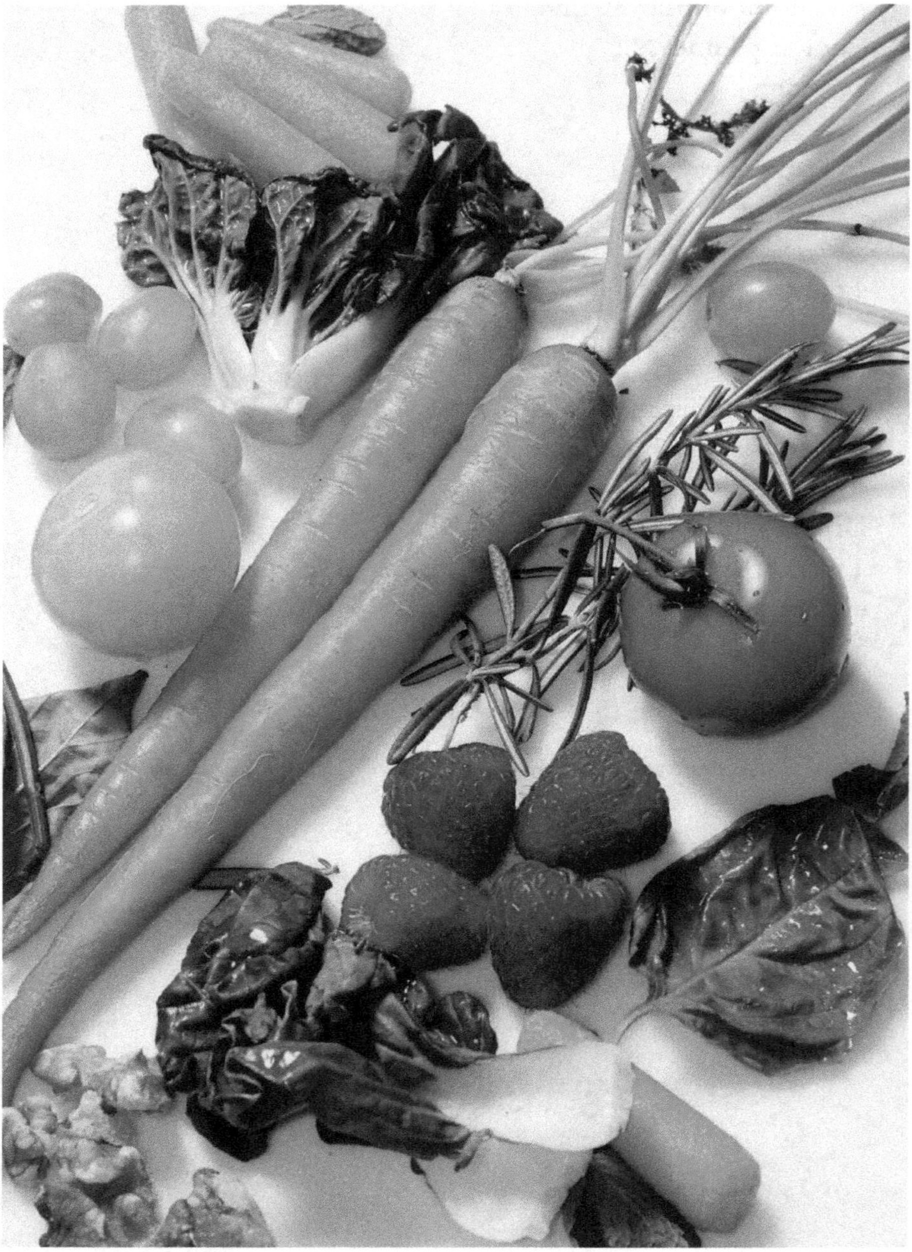

Quinoa Bowl

Preparation time: 15 minutes
Cooking Time: 15 minutes
Servings: 4

Ingredients:
1 cup quinoa
2 cups of water
1 cup tomatoes, diced
1 cup sweet pepper, diced
½ cup of rice, cooked
1 tablespoon lemon juice
½ teaspoon lemon zest, grated
1 tablespoon olive oil

Directions:
Mix up water and quinoa and cook it for 15 minutes. Then remove it from the heat and leave to rest for 10 minutes. Transfer the cooked quinoa in the big bowl. Add tomatoes, sweet pepper, rice, lemon juice, lemon zest, and olive oil. Stir the mixture well and transfer in the serving bowls.

Nutrition: Calories 290, Protein 8.4g, Carbohydrates 49.9g, Fat 6.4g, Fiber 4.3g, Cholesterol 0mg, Sodium 11mg, Potassium 435mg

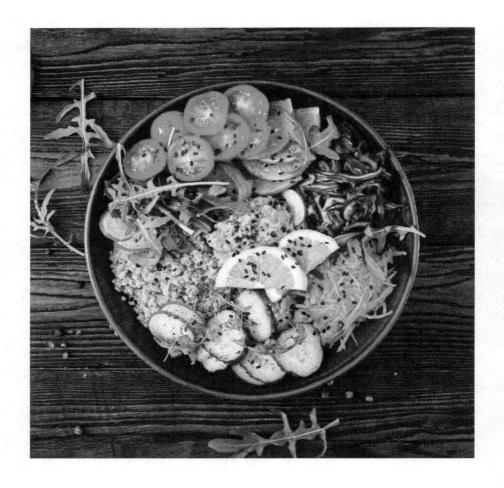

Vegan Meatloaf

Preparation time: 10 minutes
Cooking Time: 30 minutes
Servings: 6

Ingredients:
1 cup chickpeas, cooked
1 onion, diced
1 tablespoon ground flax seeds
½ teaspoon chili flakes
1 tablespoon coconut oil
½ cup carrot, diced
½ cup celery stalk, chopped
1 tablespoon tomato paste

Directions:
Heat up coconut oil in the saucepan. Add carrot, onion, and celery stalk. Cook the vegetables for 8 minutes or until they are soft. Then add chickpeas, chili flakes, and ground flax seeds. Blend the mixture until smooth with the help of the immersion blender. Then line the loaf mold with baking paper and transfer the blended mixture inside. Flatten it well and spread with tomato paste. Bake the meatloaf in the preheated to 365F oven for 20 minutes.

Nutrition: Calories 162, Protein 7.1g, Carbohydrates 23.9g, Fat 4.7g, Fiber 7g, Cholesterol 0mg, Sodium 25mg, Potassium 407mg

Seemingly Easy Portobello Mushrooms

Preparation time: 10 minutes
Cooking Time: 10 minutes
Servings: 4

Ingredients:
12 cherry tomatoes
2 ounces scallions
4 portabella mushrooms
4 1/4 ounces almond butter
Sunflower seeds and pepper to taste

Directions:
Take a large skillet and melt almond butter over medium heat.
Add mushrooms and sauté for 3 minutes.
Stir in cherry tomatoes and scallions.
Sauté for 5 minutes.
Season accordingly.
Sauté until veggies are tender.
Enjoy!

Nutrition: Calories: 154, Fat: 10g, Carbohydrates: 2g, Protein: 7g

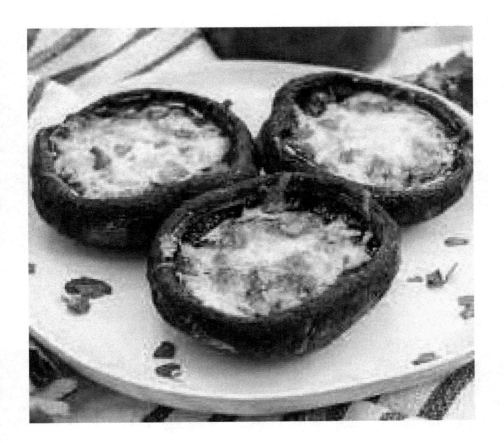

The Garbanzo Bean Extravaganza

Preparation time: 10 minutes
Cooking Time: 20 minutes
Servings: 5

Ingredients:
1 can garbanzo beans, chickpeas
1 tablespoon olive oil
1 teaspoon sunflower seeds
1 teaspoon garlic powder
1/2 teaspoon paprika

Directions:
Preheat your oven to 375 degrees F.
Line a baking sheet with a silicone baking mat.
Drain and rinse garbanzo beans, pat garbanzo beans dry and put into a large bowl.
Toss with olive oil, sunflower seeds, garlic powder, and paprika and mix well.
Spread over a baking sheet.
Bake for 20 minutes.
Turn chickpeas so they are roasted well.
Place back in oven and bake for another 25 minutes at 375 degrees F.
Let them cool and enjoy!

Nutrition: Calories: 395, Fat: 7g, Carbohydrates: 52g, Protein: 35

Hasselback Eggplant

Preparation time: 15 minutes
Cooking time: 25 minutes
Servings: 2

Ingredients:
2 eggplants, trimmed
2 tomatoes, sliced
1 tablespoon low-fat yogurt
1 teaspoon curry powder
1 teaspoon olive oil

Directions:
1. Make the cuts in the eggplants in the shape of the Hasselback. Then rub the vegetables with curry powder and fill with sliced tomatoes. Sprinkle the eggplants with olive oil and yogurt and wrap in the foil (each Hasselback eggplant wrap separately). Bake the vegetables at 375F for 25 minutes.

Nutrition: Calories 188, Protein 7g, Carbohydrates 38.1g, Fat 3g, Sodium 23mg

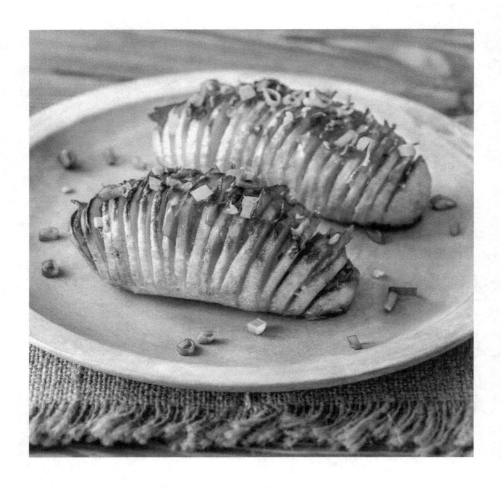

Vegetarian Kebabs

Preparation time: 15 minutes
Cooking time: 6 minutes
Servings: 4

Ingredients:
2 tablespoons balsamic vinegar
1 tablespoon olive oil
1 teaspoon dried parsley
2 tablespoons water
2 sweet peppers
2 red onions, peeled
2 zucchinis, trimmed

Directions:
1. Cut the sweet peppers and onions into medium size squares. Then slice the zucchini. String all vegetables into the skewers. After this, in the shallow bowl, mix up olive oil, dried parsley, water, and balsamic vinegar.
2. Sprinkle the vegetable skewers with olive oil mixture and transfer in the preheated to 390F grill. Cook the kebabs within 3 minutes per side or until the vegetables are light brown.

Nutrition: Calories 88, Protein 2.4g, Carbohydrates 13g, Fat 3.9g, Sodium 14mg

Corn Stuffed Peppers

Preparation time: 10 minutes
Cooking time: 35 minutes
Servings: 4

Ingredients:
4 red or green bell peppers
1 tablespoon olive oil
¼ cup onion, chopped
1 green bell pepper, chopped
2 1/2 cups fresh corn kernels
1/8 teaspoon chili powder
2 tablespoons chopped fresh parsley
3 egg whites
1/2 cup skim milk
1/2 cup water

Directions:
Prepare the oven to 350 F to preheat. Layer a baking dish with cooking spray. Cut the bell peppers from the top and remove their seeds from inside. Put the peppers in your prepared baking dish with their cut side up. Add oil to a skillet, then heat it on medium flame. Stir in onion, corn, and green pepper. Sauté for 5 minutes. Add cilantro and chili powder. Switch the heat to low. Mix milk plus egg whites in a bowl. Pour this mixture into the skillet and cook for 5 minutes while stirring. Divide this mixture into each pepper. Add some water to the baking dish. Cover the stuffed peppers with an aluminum sheet. Bake for 15 minutes, then serves warm.

Nutrition: Calories 197, Fat 5 g, Sodium 749 mg, Carbs 29 g, Protein 9 g

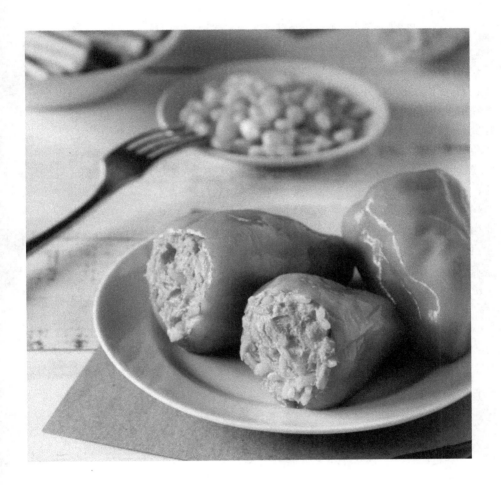

Stuffed Eggplant Shells

Preparation time: 10 minutes
Cooking time: 25 minutes
Servings: 2

Ingredients:
1 medium eggplant
1 cup of water
1 tablespoon olive oil
4 oz. cooked white beans
1/4 cup onion, chopped
1/2 cup red, green, or yellow bell peppers, chopped
1 cup canned unsalted tomatoes
1/4 cup tomatoes liquid
1/4 cup celery, chopped
1 cup fresh mushrooms, sliced
3/4 cup whole-wheat breadcrumbs
Freshly ground black pepper, to taste

Directions:

Prepare the oven to 350 degrees F to preheat. Grease a baking dish with cooking spray and set it aside. Trim and cut the eggplant into half, lengthwise. Scoop out the pulp using a spoon and leave the shell about ¼ inch thick. Place the shells in the baking dish with their cut side up. Add water to the bottom of the dish. Dice the eggplant pulp into cubes and set them aside. Add oil to an iron skillet and heat it over medium heat. Stir in onions, peppers, chopped eggplant, tomatoes, celery, mushrooms, and tomato juice. Cook for 10 minutes on simmering heat, then stirs in beans, black pepper, and breadcrumbs. Divide this mixture into the eggplant shells. Cover the shells with a foil sheet and bake for 15 minutes. Serve warm.

Nutrition: Calories 334, Fat 10 g, Sodium 142 mg, Carbs 35 g, Protein 26 g

Side Dishes – Salads - Appetizers

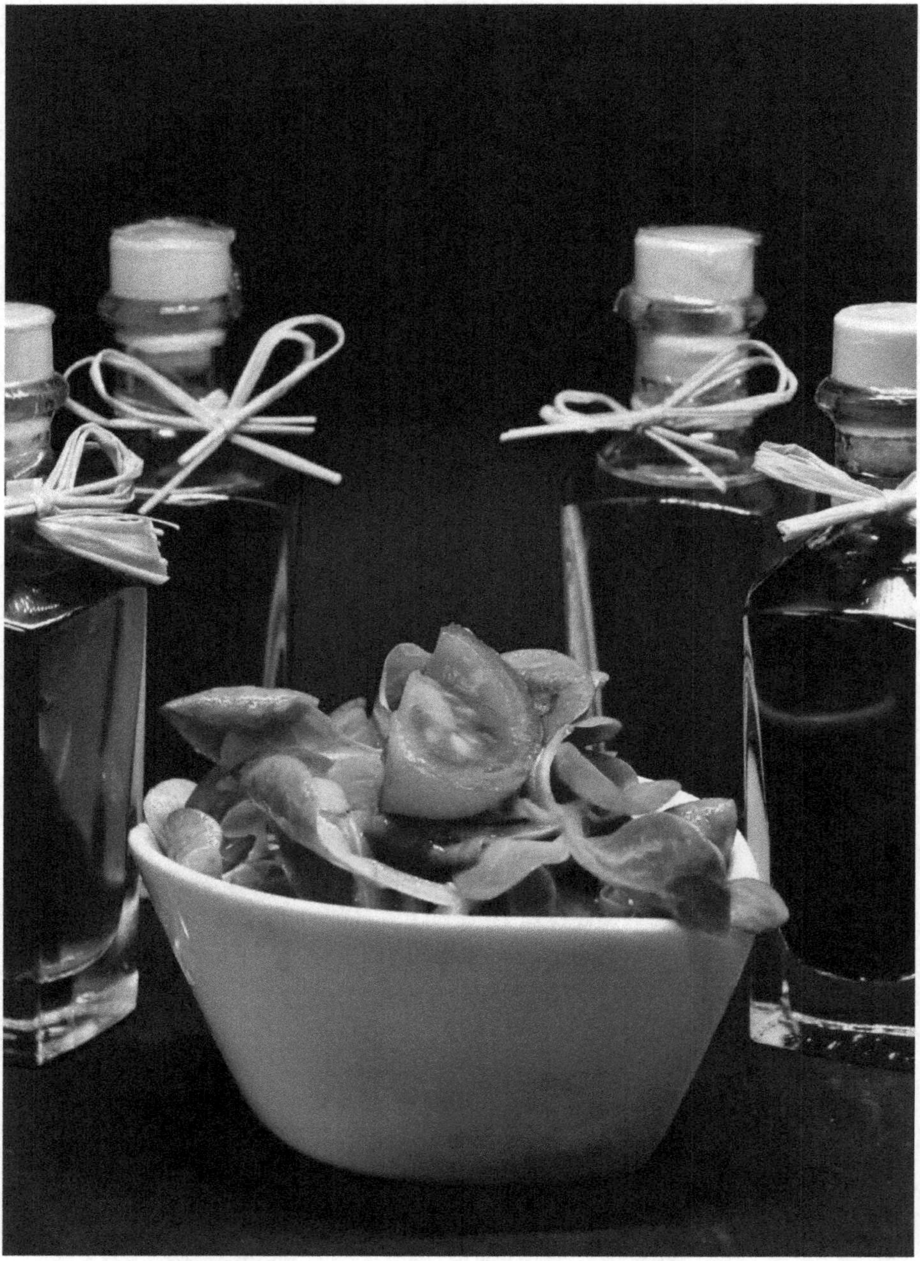

Healthy Vegetable Fried Rice

Preparation time: 5 minutes
Cooking Time: 10 minutes
Servings: 4

Ingredients:
For The Sauce:
⅓ cup garlic vinegar
1½ tablespoons dark molasses
1 teaspoon onion powder
For The Fried Rice:
1 teaspoon olive oil
2 whole eggs plus
4 egg whites, lightly beaten
1 cup frozen mixed vegetables
1 cup frozen edamame
2 cups cooked brown rice

Directions:
To make the sauce Prepare the sauce by combining the garlic vinegar, molasses, and onion powder in a glass jar. Shake well.
To make the fried rice 1. Heat oil in a large wok or skillet over medium-high heat. Add eggs and egg whites and let cook until the eggs are set (about 1 minute). Break eggs into small pieces with a spatula or. Add frozen mixed vegetables and frozen edamame. Cook for 4 minutes, stirring frequently. 2. Add the brown rice and sauce to the vegetable-and-egg mixture. Cook for 5 minutes or until heated through. 3. Serve immediately.

Nutrition: Total Calories: 210, Total Fat: 6g, Saturated Fat: 1g, Cholesterol: 93mg, Sodium: 113mg, Potassium: 183mg, Total Carbohydrates: 28g, Fiber: 3g, Sugars: 6g, Protein: 13g

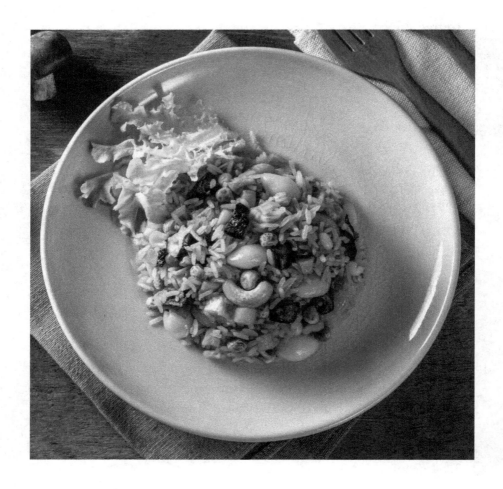

Portobello-Mushroom Cheeseburgers

Preparation time: 5 minutes
Cooking Time: 10 minutes
Servings: 4

Ingredients:
4 Portobello mushrooms, caps removed and brushed clean
1 tablespoon olive oil
½ teaspoon freshly ground black pepper
1 tablespoon red wine vinegar
4 slices reduced-fat Swiss cheese, sliced thin
4 whole-wheat 100-calorie sandwich thins
½ avocado, sliced thin

Directions:
1. Heat a skillet or grill pan over medium-high heat. Clean the mushrooms and remove the stems. Brush each cap with olive oil and sprinkle with black pepper. Place in skillet, cap-side up and cook for about 4 minutes. Flip and cook for another 4 minutes.
2. Sprinkle with the red wine vinegar and turn over. Add the cheese and cook for 2 more minutes. For optimal melting, place a lid loosely over the pan.
3. Toast the sandwich thins. Create your burgers by topping each with sliced avocado.
4. Enjoy immediately.

Nutrition: Total Calories: 245, Total Fat: 12g, Saturated Fat: 3g, Cholesterol: 15mg, Sodium: 266mg, Potassium: 507mg, Total Carbohydrates: 28g, Fiber: 8g, Sugars: 4g, Protein: 14g

Whole-Wheat Couscous Salad with Citrus and Cilantro

Preparation time: 15 minutes
Cooking time: 2 minutes
Servings: 6

Ingredients:
11/2 cups water
1 cup whole-wheat couscous
1 medium cucumber, slice in halve
1-pint grape or cherry tomatoes halved
1 jalapeño pepper, minced
2 shallots, minced
2 scallions, sliced
2 cloves garlic, minced
2 tablespoons freshly squeezed lemon juice
2 tablespoons freshly squeezed lime juice
1 teaspoon olive oil
1/4 cup chopped fresh cilantro
Freshly ground black pepper, to taste

Directions:
Mix water into a saucepan and boil over high heat. Once boiling, stir in the couscous, reduce heat to medium-low, cover, and simmer for 2 minutes. Remove pot from heat, remove the lid, and fluff couscous with a fork. Set aside to cool for 5 minutes. Scrape out the cucumber's seeds using a spoon, then dice and place into a mixing bowl. Put the rest of the fixing in the bowl along with the cooked couscous and toss well to coat. Flavor with freshly ground black pepper, then serve immediately.

Nutrition: Calories: 126, Fat: 2 g, Protein: 4 g, Sodium: 5 mg, Fiber: 2 g, Carbohydrates: 24 g, Sugar: 3 g

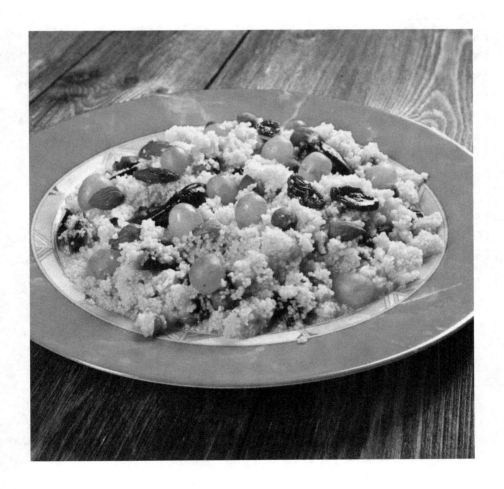

Salad Niçoise

Preparation time: 15 minutes
Cooking time: 35 minutes
Servings: 2

Ingredients:
1 small head butter lettuce
1 small cucumber
2 medium red potatoes
1 tablespoon white distilled vinegar
2 eggs
1 bunch fresh green beans, trimmed
2 tablespoons olive oil
2 tablespoons red wine vinegar
1 teaspoon salt-free prepared mustard
1 clove garlic, minced
1/2 teaspoon freshly ground black pepper
2 small tomatoes, quartered
1 (5-ounce) can no-salt-added tuna in water, drained

Directions:

Rip-up the lettuce leaves into small pieces and set aside. Peel the cucumber, halve lengthwise, and remove seeds using a spoon. Slice and set aside. Boil the potatoes into a pan with water over high heat, reduce heat slightly, and simmer until tender, about 20 minutes. Once cooked, dice, toss with white vinegar and set aside. Boil the eggs into a saucepan, with enough water to cover over high heat within 12 minutes. Once cooked, carefully crack, peel, and slice into quarters. Set aside. Boil a small pot of water, then once it's boiling, add the green beans and cook for 2 minutes. Remove beans from the pot and immediately place them in a bowl of ice water. Set aside. In a small bowl, add the oil, vinegar, mustard, garlic, and pepper and whisk well to combine. Assemble the salad on a platter, placing lettuce on the bottom and then grouping the cucumber, potatoes, eggs, green beans, tomatoes, and tuna on top. Drizzle the dressing evenly over the salad. Serve immediately.

Nutrition: Calories: 471, Fat: 20 g, Protein: 30 g, Sodium: 111 mg, Fiber: 7 g, Carbohydrates: 41 g, Sugar: 5 g

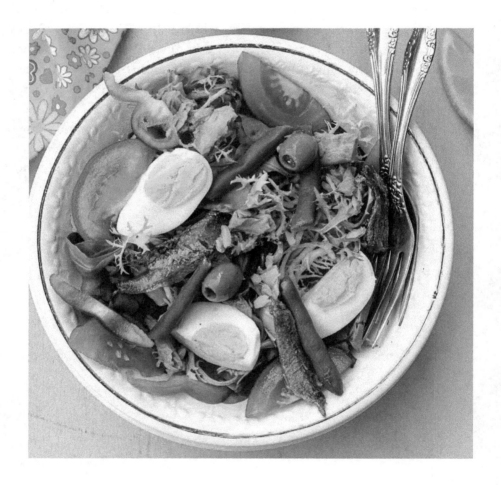

Egg and Bean Medley

Preparation time: 5 minutes
Cooking time: 18 minutes
Servings: 2

Ingredients:
½ a cup of milk
5 beaten eggs
½ a cup of tomato sauce
1 cup of cooked up white beans
2 chopped up cloves of garlic
1 teaspoon of chili powder

Directions:
Pour milk and eggs to a bowl and mix well
Add the rest of the ingredients and mix well
Stir in 1 cup of water to the pot
Transfer the bowl to your pot and lock up the lid
Cook on HIGH pressure for 18 minutes
Release the pressure naturally over 10 minutes
Serve with warm bread
Enjoy!

Nutrition: 206 Calories 9g, Fat 23g, Carbohydrates 9g, Protein 181 mg, Potassium 70mg, Sodium 112 mg

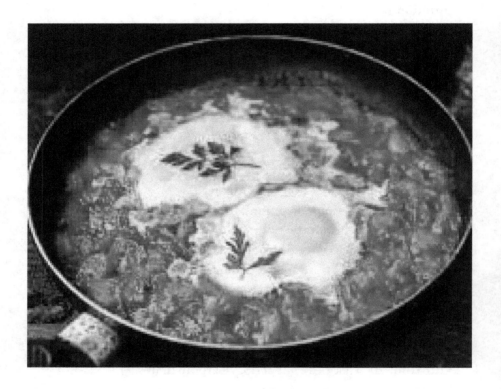

Garlic and Chive "Mash"

Preparation time: 8 minutes
Cooking time: 8 minutes
Servings: 2

Ingredients:
2 cups of vegetable stock
2 pound of peeled Yukon potatoes
4 cloves of peeled garlic
½ a cup of almond milk
½ a teaspoon of flavored vinegar ¼ cup of chives chopped up

Directions:
Add broth, garlic and potatoes to the Instant Pot
Lock up the lid and cook on HIGH pressure for 9 minutes Release the pressure naturally over 10 minutes
Drain just the amount of liquid required to maintain your required consistency
Mash the potatoes and stir in flavored vinegar and milk
Stir in chives and serve
Enjoy!

Nutrition: 293 Calories, 14g Fat 35g, Carbohydrates 8g, Protein 122mg, Potassium 81mg, Sodium 114mg

Salmon Spread

Preparation time: 10 minutes
Cooking time: 0 minutes
Servings: 4

Ingredients:
2 tablespoons horseradish
8 ounces low-fat cream cheese
2 tablespoons dill, chopped
¼ pound smoked salmon, chopped A pinch of black pepper

Directions:
In a bowl, combine the horseradish with the cream cheese, dill, salmon and black pepper, stir well and serve as a party spread.
Enjoy!

Nutrition: calories 212, fat 3, fiber 6, carbs 14, protein 7

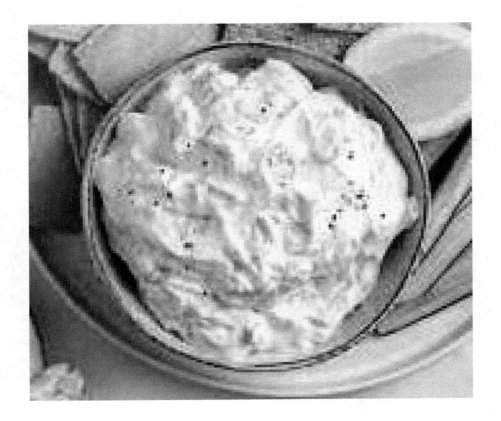

Turkey Wraps

Preparation time: 10 minutes
Cooking time: 0 minutes
Servings: 2

Ingredients:
1 peach, cut into 8 wedges
3 ounces turkey breast, cooked and cut into 8 pieces

Directions:
Roll 2 peach wedges in 2 slices of turkey, wrap, secure with a toothpick, repeat with the rest of the peach wedges and turkey and serve as a snack.
Enjoy!

Nutrition: calories 200, fat 2, fiber 5, carbs 13, protein 9

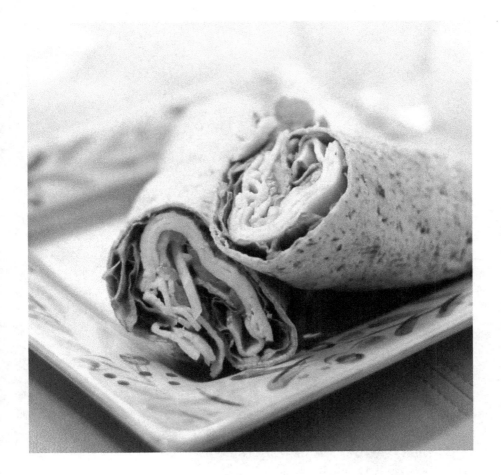

Dessert and Snacks

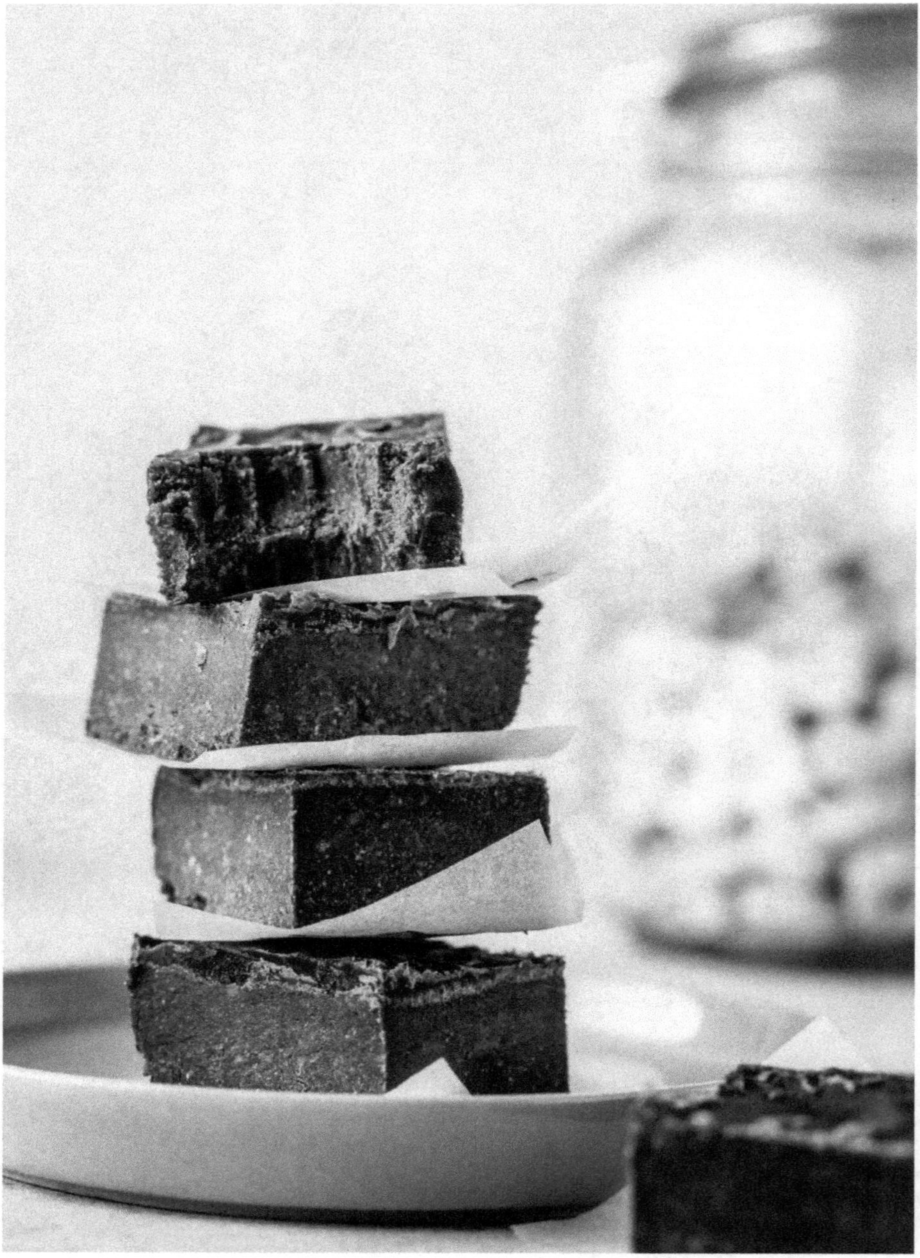

Cashew Lemon Fudge

Preparation time: 2 hours
Cooking time: 0 minutes
Servings: 4

Ingredients:
1/3 cup natural cashew butter
1 and ½ tablespoons coconut oil, melted
2 tablespoons coconut butter
5 tablespoons lemon juice
½ teaspoon lemon zest
1 tablespoons coconut sugar

Directions:
In a bowl, mix cashew butter with coconut butter, oil, lemon juice, lemon zest and sugar and stir well
Line a muffin tray with some parchment paper, scoop 1 tablespoon of lemon fudge mix in a lined muffin tray, keep in the fridge for 2 hours and serve
Enjoy!

Nutrition: calories 142, fat 4, fiber 4, carbs 8, protein 5

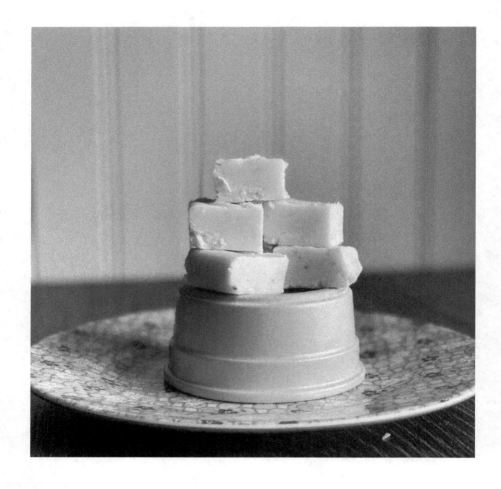

Cinnamon Peach Cobbler

Preparation time: 10 minutes
Cooking time: 4 hours
Servings: 4

Ingredients:
4 cups peaches, peeled and sliced
Cooking spray
¼ cup coconut sugar
1 and ½ cups whole wheat sweet crackers, crushed
½ cup almond milk
½ teaspoon cinnamon powder ¼ cup stevia
1 teaspoon vanilla extract ¼ teaspoon nutmeg, ground

Directions:
In a bowl, mix peaches with sugar, cinnamon, and stir.
In a separate bowl, mix crackers with stevia, nutmeg, almond milk and vanilla extract and stir.
Spray your slow cooker with cooking spray, spread peaches on the bottom, and add the crackers mix, spread, cover and cook on Low for 4 hours.
Divide into bowls and serve.

Nutrition: Calories 249, Fat 11.4g, Cholesterol 0mg, Sodium 179mg, Carbohydrate 42.7g, Fiber 3g, Sugars 15.2g, Protein 3.5g, Potassium 366mg

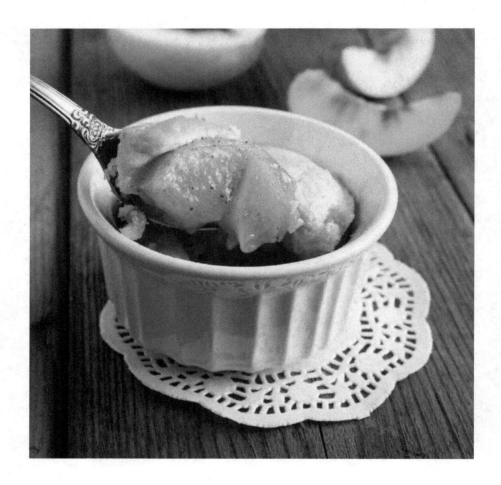

Summer Jam

Preparation time: 10 minutes
Cooking time: 3 hours
Servings: 6

Ingredients:
2 cups coconut sugar
4 cups cherries, pitted
2 tablespoons lemon juice
3 tablespoons gelatin

Directions:
In your slow cooker, mix lemon juice with gelatin, cherries and coconut sugar, stir, cover, cook on High for 3 hours, divide into bowls and serve cold.

Nutrition: Calories 171, Fat 0.1g, Cholesterol 0mg, Sodium 41mg, Carbohydrate 37.2g, Fiber 0.7g, Sugars 0.1g, Protein 3.8g, Potassium 122mg

Cinnamon Pudding

Preparation time: 10 minutes
Cooking time: 5 hours
Servings: 4

Ingredients:
2 cups white rice
1 cup coconut sugar
2 cinnamon sticks
6 and ½ cups water
½ cup coconut, shredded

Directions:
In your slow cooker, mix water with the rice, sugar, cinnamon and coconut, stir, cover, cook on High for 5 hours, discard cinnamon, divide pudding into bowls and serve warm.

Nutrition: Calories 400, Fat 4g, Cholesterol 0mg, Sodium 28mg, Carbohydrate 81.2g, Fiber 2.7g, Sugars 0.8g, Protein 7.2g, Potassium 151mg

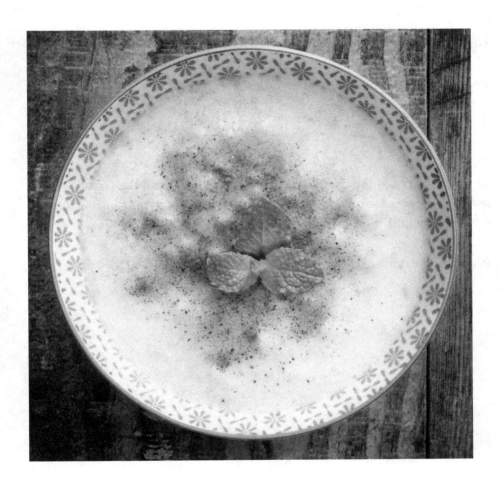

Cherry Stew

Preparation time: 10 minutes
Cooking time: 10 minutes
Servings: 6

Ingredients:
½ cup cocoa powder
1 pound cherries, pitted
¼ cup coconut sugar
2 cups water

Directions:
In a pan, combine the cherries with the water, sugar and the cocoa powder, stir, cook over medium heat for 10 minutes, divide into bowls and serve cold. Enjoy!

Nutrition: calories 207, fat 1, fiber 3, carbs 8, protein 6

Walnut Apple Mix

Preparation time: 10 minutes
Cooking time: 4 hours
Servings: 4

Ingredients:
6 big apples, roughly chopped
Cooking spray
½ cup almond flour
½ cup walnuts, chopped
¼ cup coconut oil,
melted 2 teaspoons lemon juice
3 tablespoons stevia
¼ teaspoon ginger, grated
¼ teaspoon cinnamon powder

Directions:
Spray your slow cooker with cooking spray.
In a bowl, mix stevia with lemon juice, ginger, apples and cinnamon, stir and pour into your slow cooker.
In another bowl, mix flour with walnuts and oil, stir, pour into the slow cooker, cover, and cook on Low for 4 hours.
Divide into bowls and serve.

Nutrition: Calories 474, Fat 30.3g, Cholesterol 0mg, Sodium 9mg, Carbohydrate 58.4g, Fiber 10.7g, Sugars 35g, Protein 7.7g, Potassium 444mg

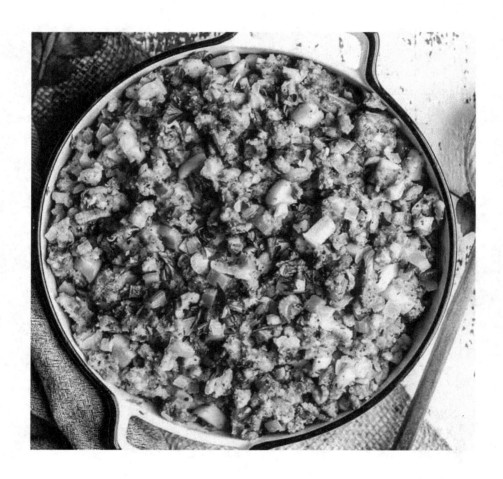

Authentic Medjool Date Truffles

Preparation time: 10-15 minutes
Cooking Time: Nil
Serving: 4

Ingredients:
2 tablespoons peanut oil
½ cup popcorn kernels
1/3 cup peanuts, chopped
1/3 cup peanut almond butter
¼ cup wildflower honey

Directions:
Take a pot and add popcorn kernels, peanut oil.
Place it over medium heat and shake the pot gently until all corn has popped. Take a saucepan and add honey, gently simmer for 2-3 minutes.
Add peanut almond butter and stir.
Coat popcorn with the mixture and enjoy!

Nutrition: Calories: 430, Fat: 20g, Carbohydrates: 56g, Protein 9g

Tasty Mediterranean Peanut Almond butter Popcorns

Preparation time: 5 minutes + 20 minutes chill time
Cooking Time: 2-3 minutes
Serving: 4

Ingredients:
3 cups Medjool dates, chopped
12 ounces brewed coffee
1 cup pecans, chopped
½ cup coconut, shredded
½ cup cocoa powder

Directions:
Soak dates in warm coffee for 5 minutes.
Remove dates from coffee and mash them, making a fine smooth mixture.
Stir in remaining ingredients (except cocoa powder) and form small balls out of the mixture.
Coat with cocoa powder, serve and enjoy!

Nutrition: Calories: 265, Fat: 12g, Carbohydrates: 43g, Protein 3g

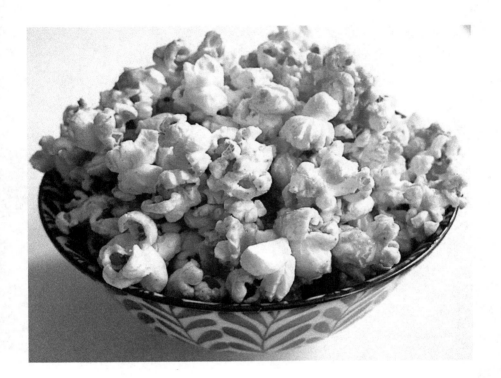